The Tai Chi Way TO BETTER BALANCE

An Illustrated Manual

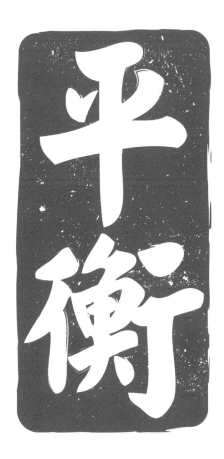

DON ETHAN MILLER
4-Time National Tai Chi Tui Shou Champion,
Creator of Tai Chi Boot Camp, Tai Chi Equipment
Training and Chen Man Ching: The Master Tapes

PRESENTED BY DAN KLEIMAN
Executive Director of Brookline Tai Chi and the
CDC-Approved Falls Prevention Program: Tai Chi
for Healthy Aging

ISBN: 978-1493592845

Table of Contents

Tai Chi Balance Training

WELCOME TO THE
TAI CHI WAY TO BETTER BALANCE

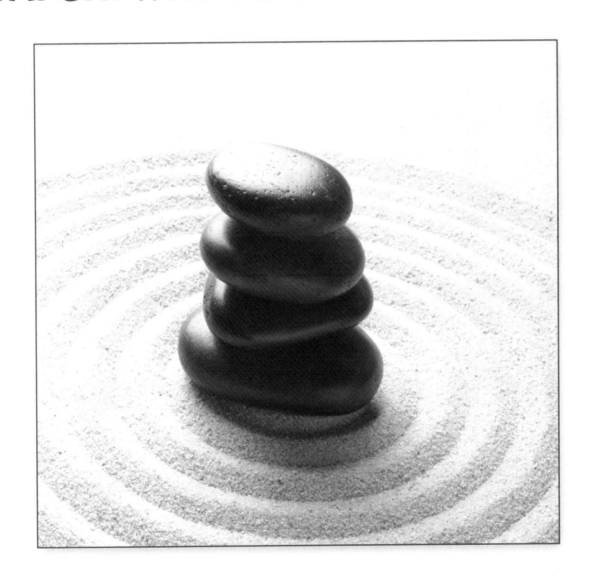

THE COST OF A FALL

Have you noticed a loved one who, in the last few years, has been less and less likely to go out? Are they moving a little slower and maybe a little stiffer too? Each year, one out of every three adults over the age of 65 has a fall. You are five times more likely to be hospitalized for a fall-related injury than an injury from any other cause. Fear of falling has a huge impact on how older adults live day to day.

The good news is that Tai Chi is emerging as one of the safest and most effective ways to regain your balance, avoid falls, and cultivate gracefulness through meditative movement.

At Brookline Tai Chi, where I have been Executive Director since 2005, we are regularly being approached by insurance companies, government agencies, and research universities to weigh in on what makes an effective Tai Chi balance training program.

Thirty years ago, when my first Tai Chi teacher, Bruce Frantzis, came back to the US to spread the Tai Chi he learned in China, he found out that many basic concepts were not being taught. Only a fraction of the vast Potential of the art was being shared. Instead of endless forms and choreography, Bruce set out to teach the Inner Form of Tai Chi.

Most people expect to learn "The Form" because what you typically see people practicing in the park every morning, but that's actually just the outer most shell of real Tai Chi. Bruce revealed the inner workings of Tai Chi, that make it so powerful for restoring health and unlocking hidden internal energy, well into old age.

Now, Tai Chi is moving into a new phase of popular understanding in the West, to serve an important public health need.

To help me share with you the real Tai Chi Way to Better Balance, I have sought out another champion of the Inner Form approach to Tai Chi, Don Ethan Miller. Don has practiced and taught Tai Chi for more than 40 years, won national titles in Tai Chi Push Hands Sparring and has, in my opinion, a unique, direct, and profound approach to Tai Chi education.

Simple, Yet Profound

The exercises you will discover in this program may seem simple at first. They are accessible to almost any level of physical fitness and balance. In fact, the exercises are precisely layered to allow almost anyone to regain their balance safely and gradually.

Layers of Progress

As you work through the levels in the book, you'll notice that the skills you build are layered one on top of the next.

First you get comfortable on two legs, with no distractions. But what happens when you only have one leg to stand on? Or you add an arm motion and a head turn? Slowly, you will add layers, and each time, you will understand how the new layer makes you stronger, more stable, and more internally connected in accordance with the Tai Chi principles you will learn about in the next section.

As the complexity of the exercises increase, so will your rate of discovery. We see people burst out of classes all the time. They can't wait to bounce down the street or frolic in the park. It's kind of goofy when you their eyes light up like little kids again!

And that's what I wish for you and hope we can share with the world about the Tai Chi Way to Better Balance.

Now, on to the balance training,

Dan Kleiman

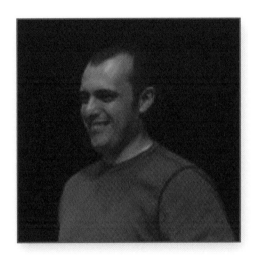

Dan Kleiman is the Executive Director of Brookline Tai Chi where he leads the CDC-approved Tai Chi for Healthy Aging Program, focused on falls prevention for seniors.

FROM THE AUTHOR

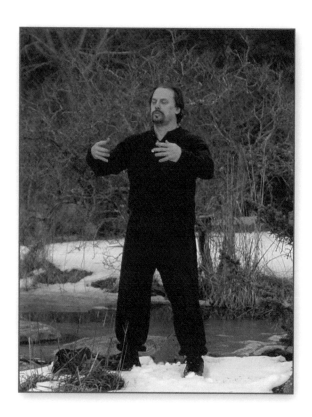

My first Tai Chi lesson, over forty years ago, was about balance. I was a young, strong Black Belt in Korean Karate, and I had brought my class to visit a 70 year old Tai Chi master T.T.Liang, whom I had heard was teaching the then very little known art just a few hours from us. He seemed a kind, intelligent man with a twinkle in his eyes. He raised his arm in front of his body and invited me to push him. I put both brick-breaking hands on his forearm and pushed forward forcefully. Liang relaxed his arm, withdrew his body slightly, and turned his waist — and I stumbled forward into the empty space he had created, almost falling on my face. He smiled, I laughed, he laughed with me.

It was the beginning of a beautiful friendship, and a lifetime of Tai Chi.

The exercises contained in this book represent the distillation of my four decades of study and practice in Tai Chi and other martial arts, specifically applied to issues of balance, equilibrium and stability-in-motion. Many of them are, as Dan says, deceptively simple. It is in the doing that you will discover their power to change your state in the direction of not only improved physical balance, but greater naturalness, vitality, and psychological well-being.

I encourage you to take the time to practice the exercises, take note of their effects (I guarantee you there will be many); and to share this program with friends and others who might benefit from it.

Please feel free to contact me at donmillertaichi@gmail.com with any questions, reports, realizations or revelations you may have.

As I like to say about my classes and workshops, "Upgrades and Laughter Guaranteed!"

With my warmest Tai Chi regards,

Don Ethan Miller

Tai Chi master-instructor and 4-time Tai Chi Tuishou National Champion.

TAI CHI AND BALANCE

Tai Chi masters are known for maintaining vitality, balance and mobility well into old age. My first Tai Chi teacher, Master T.T. Liang, lived to be 102, and in his mid-eighties was still throwing young, large guys around in the Tai Chi game — somewhat akin to upright grappling or sumo — called "push hands" (tuishou). His consummate skill with Chinese weapons — sword, cutlass, staff, spear — was still evident well into his 90's.

In the ten years I studied with him, I cannot say I ever saw Master Liang lose his balance. What is more, I learned much later that he was practicing Tai Chi on severely compromised feet, permanently damaged by the horrendous torture he endured at the hands of the Japanese during WWII.

Many other Tai Chi masters are notable for their sustained "youthfulness" of the legs and hips, supple and strong in the decades when many are becoming stiff and weak.

Some of these effects are probably the result of simply continuing to exercise and move around, in fairly complex ways, and never "retiring" from movement. But they are also, I believe, in large part the embodiment of 3 major Tai Chi

Principles that are central to the art and developed fully over many decades of practice. These Principles — Rooting, Central Equilibrium, and Yin and Yang — are critical components of attaining, maintaining, and/or regaining excellent balance, and they underlie the exercises that will be presented in this book.

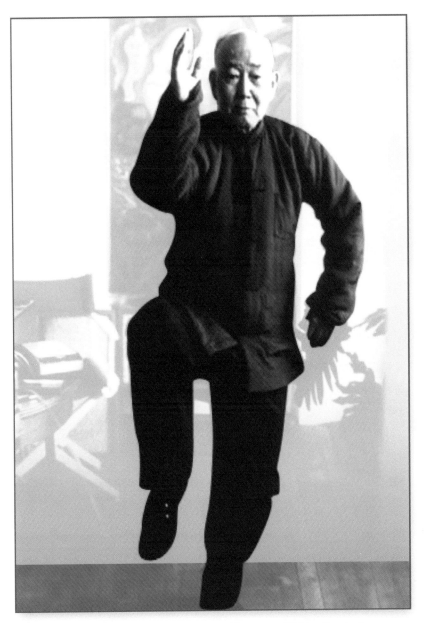

The eminent Liang T'ung T'sai, performs the Tai Chi posture "Golden Rooster," sometime in his late 80's.

Rooting

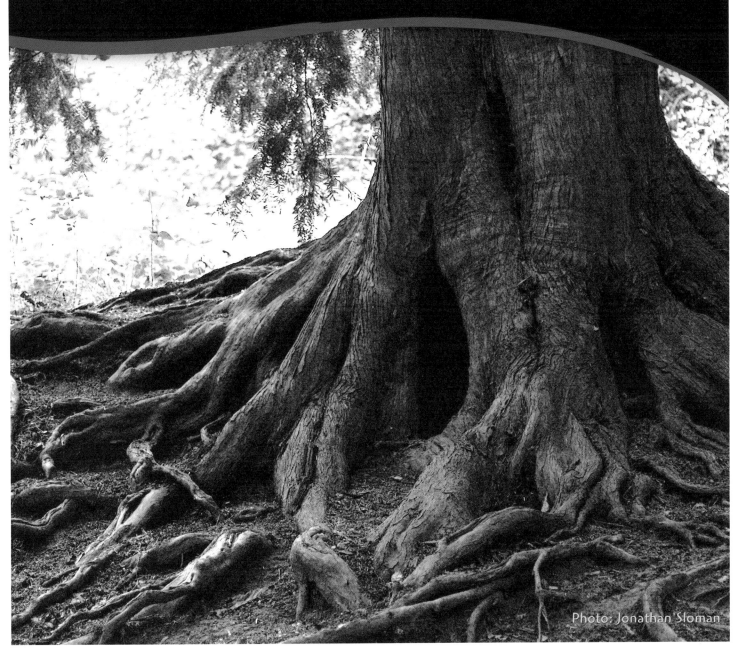

Photo: Jonathan Sloman

Rooting means connecting to the earth, not only physically but also energetically, mentally, even spiritually. In the West we have the concept of being "grounded," but Tai Chi goes further. To be rooted means that, while we do not have actual physical roots like trees or other members of the plant kingdom, some essential aspect of ourselves is intertwined with the geography we inhabit, with nature, with the magnetic core of the earth. There are specific practices which enhance and develop these qualities, and they are found in Tai Chi more than in any other art. "Without rooting, there is no Tai Chi." Someone who is rooted is not only physically but psychologically stable, less prone to being imbalanced by the winds of circumstance, emotion, stress, the constant changes of external events. Rooting gives Tai Chi its unique combination of calmness and power, strength and relaxation.

Another way to look at rooting is neurological: in modern society, for most people, the vast majority of actions and interactions are conducted using (primarily) the neuromuscular circuitry connecting the hands and arms, the eyes, the mouth and tongue, and the brain. We drive, we type, we text, we talk into smart phones, we cook meals — almost all the activities of daily life involve utilizing the circuitry to the upper quarter of the body. But we use other areas of our neural circuitry — those involving our legs, feet, torso, hips, and backs — far less than our ancestors did just a few generations ago; and remarkably less than the real "human animal" body (which evolved to its present form about 100,000 years ago) was designed for.

Rooting rectifies this imbalance, by getting us back into our feet, our legs, back, and hips, and minimizing, at least for awhile, our reliance on the eye-hand-head circuitry. In terms of simple biological functions, it is the reactivation of the natural support, propulsion, and adaptation circuitry of the whole body. We get to turn the neurological hourglass back, the way it was designed, and the result is both greater physical stability, and greater psychological balance.

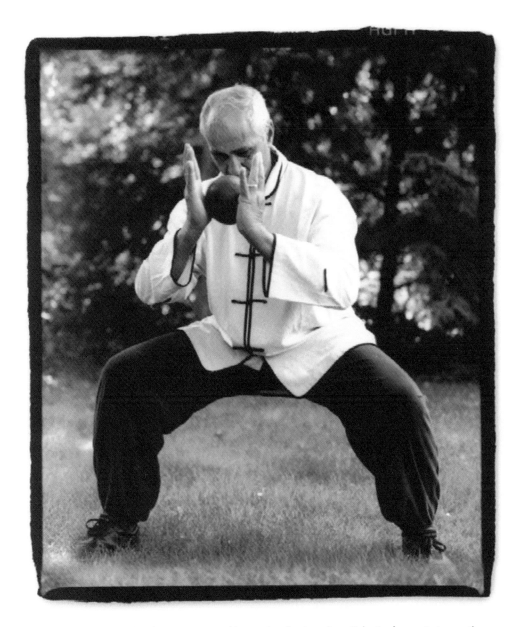

The great Willem de Thouars, master of internal and external martial arts, demonstrates rooting of body, mind, and spirit.

Central Equilibrium

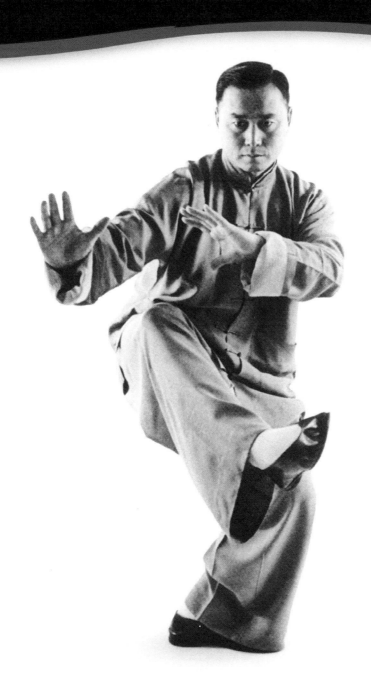

Overleaf: The magnificent Tung Hu Ling, showing perfect central equilibrium and balance of multiple elements in the Yang Tai Chi posture, "Lotus Sweep with Leg."

The basic Tai Chi idea of Central Equilibrium (Zhong Ding) is fairly simple: think of a vertical pole supported by struts or guy-wires that extend to the ground front and back, left and right, creating a balance of forces that contribute to maintaining the vertical alignment of the pole.

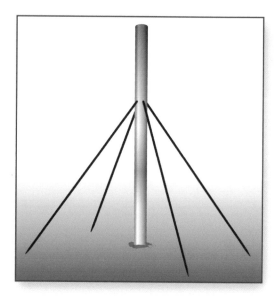

In another sense, Zhong Ding is also like a plumb line that extends in both directions, through the body's center of gravity — downwards, towards the center of the earth, along the line of gravity; and upwards along the same line, to the "heavens."

Even when the body is not standing vertically — as for example, when we fold at the hips and knees to sit into, or rise from, a chair — the Zhong Ding is like an invisible line that informs us of how our weight is distributed and organizes it around an invisible "center."

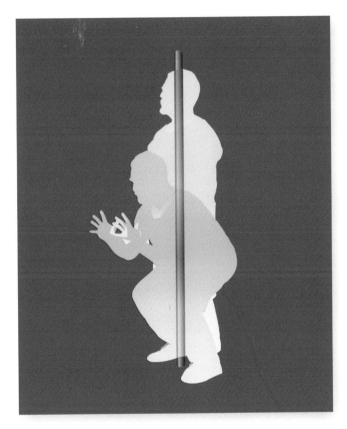

In another sense, Zhong Ding is like a gyroscope, that maintains a balance of weights and forces in three dimensions — so that, say if we are lifting a suitcase with one hand, we counterbalance the suitcase's weight with appropriate shifts and muscle contractions so that it forms a balanced whole with the rest of the body. It is, in other words, the continuous adjustment and re-adjustment of the body to maintain balance as we move or encounter objects and forces outside ourselves.

Once again, Tai Chi has special practices to enhance and develop this quality, so that no matter what our position or action, we have a base of support under our center of gravity and an integrity of the whole system that automatically adjusts to change.

Yin & Yang

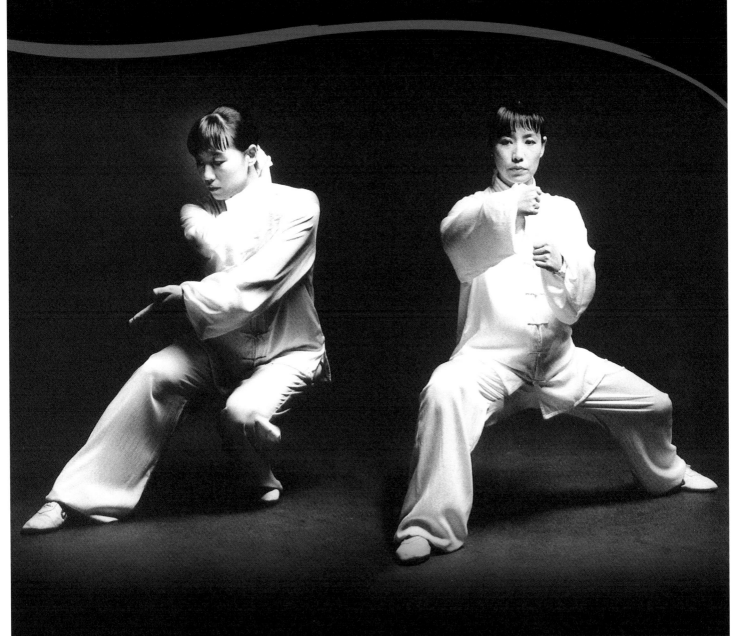

Overleaf: Master Hong Yijiao, demonstrating Yin and Yang qualities in two postures from Chen Tai Chi: the first coiled and sensitive, the second expansive and powerful.

Yin and Yang is a Taoist concept which seems superficially simple but can actually be quite profound. In Tai Chi, all phenomena can be viewed as having both Yin and Yang aspects: the Yang generally being the more positive, active, outwardly focused, aggressive (especially in the literal meaning of "going towards"), "up," bright, and overt; while the Yin generally referring to the negative, inwardly focused, passive or stable, dark, hidden, receiving, peaceful. Hard/Soft, Up/Down, Out/In, Moving/Still, Doing/Being, Figure/Ground are some common pairs of yin-yang opposites, or polarities.

In relation to physical balance, the concept of Yin and Yang is critically important. From a stationary position (yin), any movement (yang) creates a condition of imbalance. Thus it is essential to learn to balance the Yang of activity with the Yin of stillness, or wholeness — to find the state that Tai Chi refers to as "stillness within movement."

This is why many of the Tai Chi practices are done slowly, such that the practitioner actually feels equally that he or she is moving and not moving, at the same time.

From the Tai Chi perspective, all loss of balance is an error in the balance of Yin and Yang, to be corrected through training the yin and yang qualities both separately and together. For example , when we move the upper body — the trunk, head, and arms (Yang), we must balance this by moving the lower body — the hips, legs, and feet (Yin), at the same time and in the right direction and speed.

Adopting the "yin-yang" perspective is a productive way to analyze what is going on when someone has impaired function; and also to prescribe the correct exercises or practices to regain the dynamic balance of two polarities — which is the actual meaning of Tai Chi. Many of these practices will be found in the pages that follow.

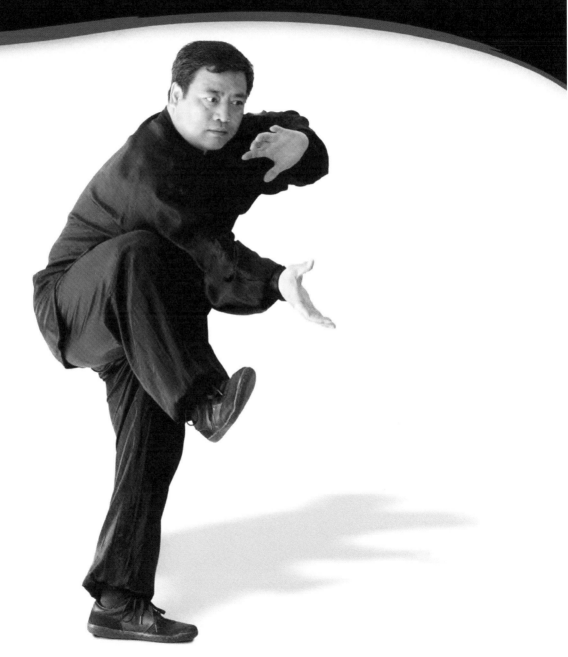

Overleaf: Master Yang Fu Kui, showing perfect balance in a dynamic pose, the fruit of his decades of training in Tai Chi, Yiquan, BaGua, and other internal martial arts.

HOW TO USE THIS BOOK

The Tai Chi Balance Training exercises that follow are designed to improve your balance through the Tai Chi principles of Rooting, Central Equilibrium, and Yin-Yang. They are progressive, systematic, reliable, and safe. Regardless of your current level of balance and physical ability, I urge you to start with the Level One practices, and progress to Levels Two, and Three only when the exercises on your current level have become easy. There is no timetable for progress, as each person is different.

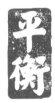 When you see this chop, the Chinese characters for Balance ("Ping Heng"), it denotes an exercise (or group of exercises) that can be practiced as a "stand-alone," which by itself will produce a significant change in your balance functions. Each of these can be practiced separately (taking only a few minutes) or combined into a full Tai Chi Balance Training routine — Level One, Two, or Three — that will take between 15 and 30 minutes to complete.

I also strongly recommend keeping track of your experiences, noting any sensations, changes, improvements etc in a notebook. This will prove extremely valuable as you progress in your Tai Chi Balance Training.

And, as with all Tai Chi and internal kung fu practices, we start and end with a simple, but profound, form of standing meditation called Wu Chi.

Wu Chi Standing

Wu Chi is a term in Tai Chi and other Chinese internal arts that is variously translated as: no limit, formless, emptiness, the Void, Infinity, Origin, primordial/original state, undivided (into Yin and Yang), etc. The standing posture called Wu Chi is one in which everything is present, yet nothing stands out; where the mind is calm and empty of thought, and the body is relaxed, upright without effort, whole. This posture forms the basis for all Tai Chi balance work, and every practice session should both begin and end with a minimum of 30 seconds to one minute of quiet Wu Chi standing.

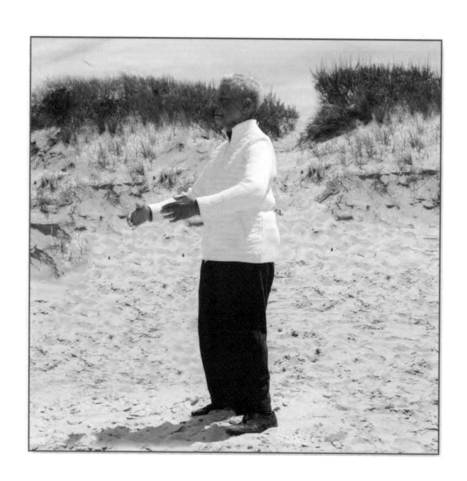

- Stand with feet shoulder width apart, feet pointing forwards. Your weight should be centered over the middle of each foot, or very slightly forwards (just behind the ball of the foot). Please do not allow the weight to skew to the heels, the toes, or the inside or outside edges of the feet.

- Your knees should be very slightly bent, not locked straight, such that you can "feel the ground" with your feet, legs, and hips. This feeling, an awareness of the lower body structure and its relation the ground, is the first and most important quality in the art of Tai Chi. It is the beginning of the process of "rooting," or "developing root," which is (in the Tai Chi perspective), not only a physical increase in stability, balance, and internal power, but an actual energetic connection to the earth itself.

- This grounding or rooting sensation does not need to be forced, or created or imposed by your mind. It is there to be experienced, simply by standing with a slight bend in the knees, ankles, and hip joints, and by directing your awareness to your legs and feet. (At some point, you may also find that you will also become aware of the area below your feet.)

- Your torso should be erect, vertical, but as relaxed as possible without slumping. There is no need to puff the chest out, or tighten the stomach muscles, or make any other adjustments other than finding a comfortable, relaxed uprightness. In Tai Chi, we often use the image of a string pulling the top of the head gently upwards. This works well for many people, but be sure not to tilt the head backwards, lifting the chin up instead of the crown of the head. If anything, there should be a slight feeling of lengthening in the back of the neck — like a kitten being carried by the scruff of the neck. But gently!

Your hands and arms can be in one of the following three positions:

1. Hanging loosely at your sides. Fingers can rest against your thighs if this is comfortable.

2. As above but with a gentle extension of the fingers (including thumbs), "opening" the hands and allowing the arms to move very slightly away from the body.

3. Arms softly rounded and held in front of the body, hands somewhere between navel and chest level, the shoulders remaining relaxed.

Your eyes should be "soft": that is, not staring, but gently looking either directly ahead or slightly downwards.

Your attention:

• At first, make sure you have the grounded, "rooted" feeling described above.

• Then, pay attention to your breathing and allow it to become naturally deep, calm, and relaxed.

• Finally, allow your mind to empty of any specific thoughts or ideas, but maintain a calm, relaxed awareness of what is occurring both inside you and all around you.

Remain in this state for the duration of the practice, which should be from a half-minute up to (as your capacity improves) 3-5 minutes or more.

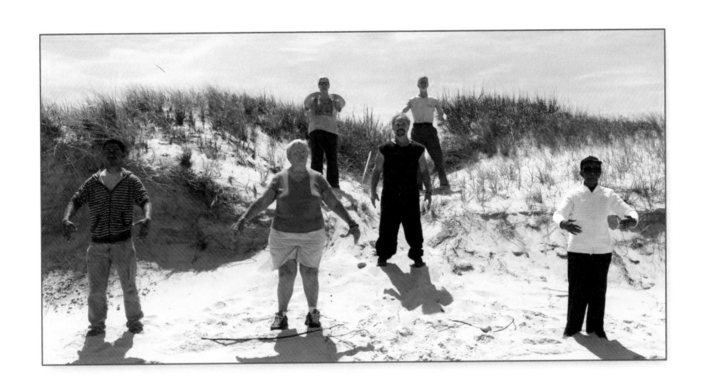

By practicing the Wu Chi posture before and after your Tai Chi balance exercises, you will get a definite sense of how the exercises are affecting your stability, spatial awareness, energy, and other factors. It is like a blank notebook on which you can record your progress. It is also a tremendous practice in its own right and one which you can utilize profitably for your entire life.

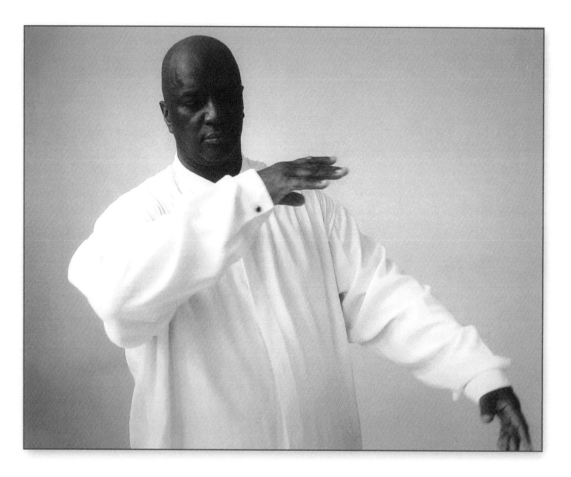

Tai Chi/Yiquan Master Arthur Goodridge shows the deeply calm, internal Wu Chi state in motion, in the Tai Chi exercise "Wave Hands In the Clouds."

Tai Chi Balance Training

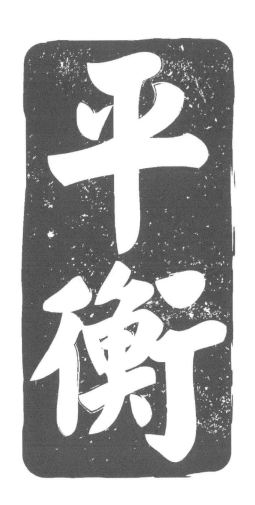

Level One

SINGLE WEIGHTING

While good balance is a combination of many factors, the ability of the body to comfortably hold its entire weight on one leg is a crucial component. Many people are "in a hurry" to get the weight off one leg, as the muscles (and the structural alignments) are simply unused to sustaining the pressure of the entire bodyweight on just one leg — leading to a hasty, imbalanced movements. In Tai Chi, we say that "the root is deeper when single weighted." The following exercises introduce the feeling of "single weighting" and build leg strength and alignment, and for many people produce a noticeable improvement in balance almost immediately.

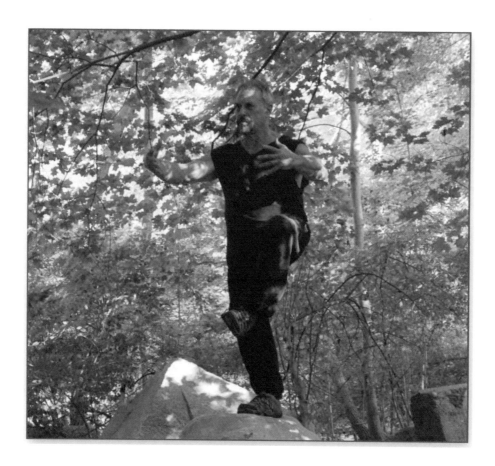

CHENG MAN CHING

Cheng Man Ching (Zheng Manqing) was one of the first true masters of Tai Chi to teach in North America, and his influence on the spread of the art in the US (as well as Taiwan, Europe, and SE Asia) is profound. Considered a "Master of 5 Excellences," he was also a world-renowned brush painter, poet, calligrapher, and physician.

The following exercise was taught by Professor Cheng as a fundamental practice for developing root. Deceptively simple and easy, if done correctly it will have a powerful effect with just a few minutes of practice. Done regularly for a month...well, try it and see for yourself!

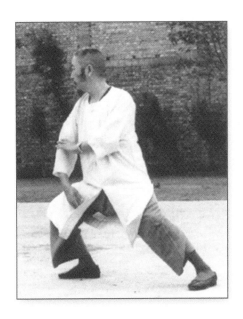

THE JOY WHICH LASTS

The joy of continuous growth, of helping to develop in ourselves and others the talents and abilities with which we were born—the gifts of heaven to mortal men. To revive the exhausted and to rejuvenate that which is in decline, so that we are enabled to dispel sickness and suffering. With the constancy of the planets in their courses or of the dragon in his cloud wrapped path, let us enter the land of health and ever after walk within its bounds. This is the joy which lasts, that we can carry with us to the end of our days. And tell me, if you can; what greater happiness can life bestow?

- Cheng Man Ching,
"Hall of Happiness"

平衡 MASTER CHENG'S SINGLE LEG ROOTING

Stand in front of a solid sturdy chair back, or a countertop, desk, or other solid surface that is approximately waist height. Place both hands (or, if you prefer, just the fingers of both hands) on the surface and keep them there for the entire exercise. (Please do not remove your hands because the exercise is "too easy.") Shift all your weight to one leg, again with the knee slightly unlocked as in the Wu Chi posture. Allow the non-weighted leg to just gently connect to the ground, preferably with just the toes touching. It is important that you get as close to 100% of the your bodyweight supported by just one leg.

In this position, relax your body as much as possible. Breathe deeply, releasing tension from your neck, shoulders, back, arms, stomach, and hips with each exhale. Feel your weight dropping deeper and deeper, through the support leg to the ankle and foot, and even through the foot into the ground. Stay on this leg as long as is comfortable, without straining; then switch to the other leg. Repeat on each leg 3 times, preferably for 30 seconds to one minute each time. (Your time will depend on your capacity; but you will find that the exercise becomes much easier after only a handful or sessions.)

After 3 "rounds," return to the basic 2-leg standing position, and note any changes in how you feel. Now, walk a little, also noting any difference. You can repeat this process several times throughout a single day.

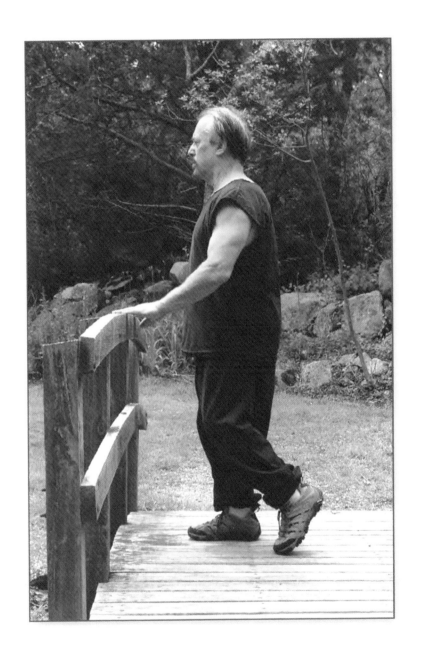

UNIVERSAL POST

Once you are comfortable with the first exercise, you can move on to the following single-weighting practice, called "The Universal Post":

Stand with the weight 85-95% on one leg, with the supporting knee very slightly bent, ie, just an inch or a few few inches lower than the "locked" position. Touch the ball and toes of the other foot to the ground, about one foots-length in front and slightly to the side. The angle between the two feet should be around 45 degrees.

The front foot is primarily a balance point, but should not carry any of the main bodyweight.

The arms can be in any of the 3 following positions:

1. Down at the sides, held slightly away from the body;
2. At waist height, palms down; or
3. At chest height, arms rounded in front of you, "as if embracing a tree."

Relax as much as possible, breathe deeply and calmly, and maintain this position for 30 seconds to one minute; then change sides and repeat on the other leg. As you get better at it, you can do 2-5 rounds of holding on each side; or you can progress to holding for 2-3 minutes, once only, on each leg.

As with all Tai Chi balance exercises, finish by returning to the Wu Chi position briefly, and appreciate how much more stable you have become.

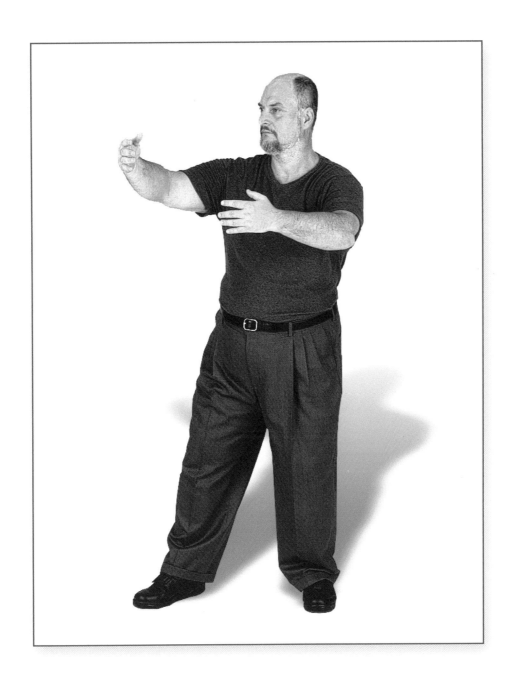

Tai Chi/Qigong/BaGua Master Bruce Frantzis shows Central Equilibrium and calm power in Universal Post. Photo by Guy Hearn.

TWO-LEG STANCE CHALLENGES

While most people can hold the basic Wu Chi Posture fairly comfortably for a minute or more (if you can not, this should be your entire practice), as soon as movements of the hands and arms, the eyes, head and neck, hips or torso, are introduced, or required by circumstance — such as, turning to look at the source of a sudden loud noise, or reaching to get something from a high shelf — the "degree of difficulty" in maintaining a balanced posture goes up abruptly. In the Tai Chi Balance Training Program, we introduce such challenges slowly and deliberately, allowing the body to adapt to the changes in position and weight distribution correctly and without making any "mistakes."

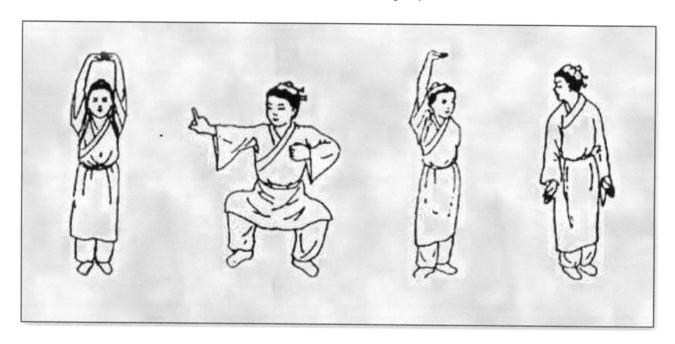

MOVING ONE ARM

- Stand with weight even on both feet, knees unlocked as in Wu Chi posture, above.

- Slowly, move one arm up and around in a smooth circle. Repeat several times, in both directions.

- Now, move the hand and arm in more complex patterns, as if drawing lines and shapes in the air.

- As you do this, keep at least 50% of your awareness in your legs, feet, and torso, so that the arm movements are "countered," or balanced, by changes in the rest of the body.

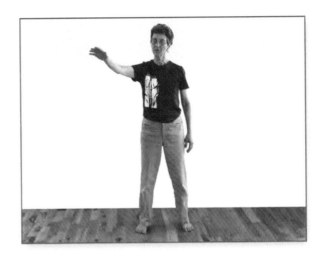

- Repeat with the other hand/arm. Experiment to see how far you can move the arm in various directions while staying balanced and rooted in your legs.

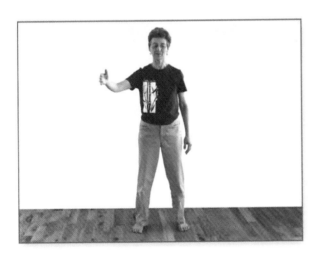

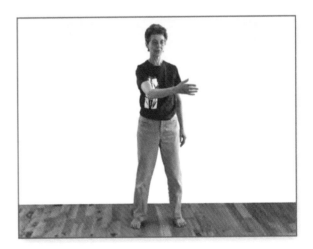

LOOKING TO
LEFT AND RIGHT

• Start in the basic Wu Chi stance, arms at your sides.

• Slowly, turn to look 45 degrees to one side — allowing the torso to twist gently to support the movement

• FOR SAFETY AND STABILITY, do not just move the head while keeping the body immobile; conversely, do not twist the legs in such a way that you torque your knees and lose the stability of the stance.

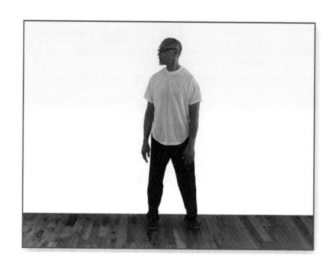

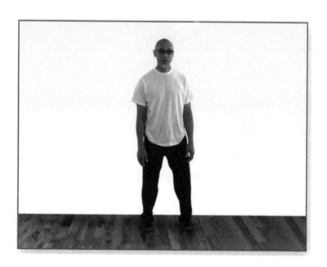

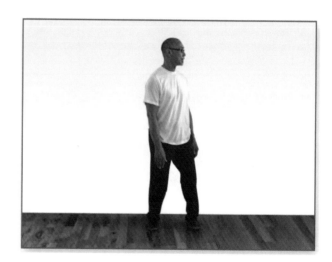

MOVING BOTH ARMS

Stand as above, but now experiment with slowly moving both arms in a variety of patterns:

- circling the hands clockwise and counterclockwise in front of the body

- circling from in to out and out to in in front of the body

- creating more complex patterns of movement in front, to the side, above and behind the body

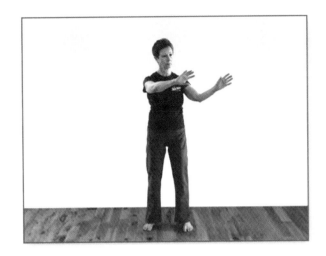

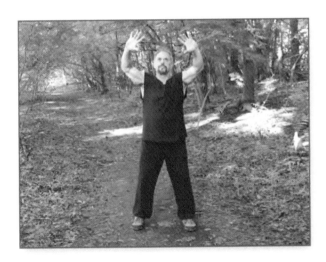

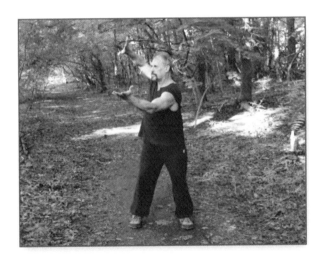

In all cases, keep half your awareness in the feet, legs, and torso, to "ground" and stabilize your whole body during the arm/hand movements. We are balancing the Yang of movement with the Yin of stillness.

SWINGING THE ARMS

This exercise increases the challenges by adding greater speed and momentum. Start in the grounded, rooted position. Swing your arms, letting them feel loose and somewhat heavy, in three patterns that follow.

Allow the torso to move in support of all these motions, so they are not occurring just from the shoulders down. Maintain the grounded, rooted Tai Chi quality and keep half your attention on your stance.

Backwards and forwards, as if walking:

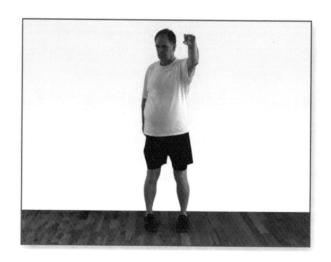

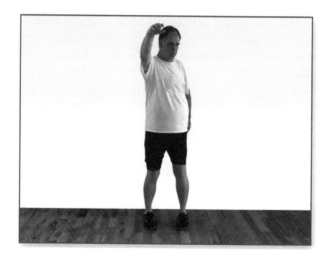

Up and down, both hands moving together:

Turning left and right by twisting the torso:

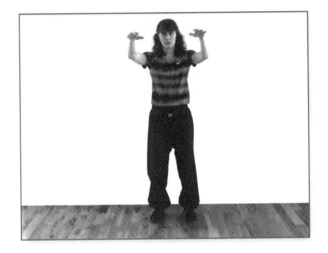

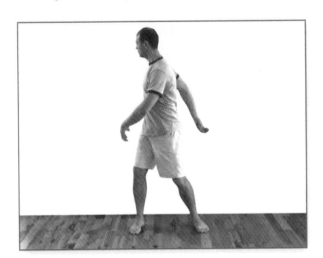

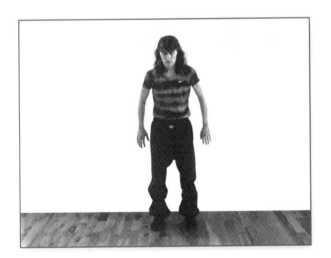

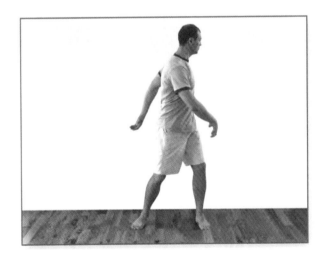

HOLDING AN OBJECT WITH ONE HAND

Stand in the basic two-leg stance while holding an object with some weight to it (minimally, a can of peas or beans; maximally, a filled small suitcase — ie, between 1 and 25 pounds) in one hand.

- Hold for 15-30 seconds, feeling your body adapt to the weight of the object to maintain equilibrium.

- Put the object down (on a chair or table if it is difficult to place on the floor);

- Then pick up with the other hand and repeat the adaptation.

- For a larger challenge, try transferring the object slowly from one hand to the other.

- Experiment with objects of different shapes and sizes. Pay attention to your balance and your connection to the ground as you work with different objects.

- After each hold (both sides), stand without anything and feel the effects.

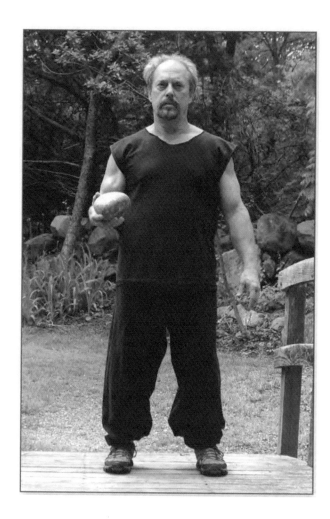

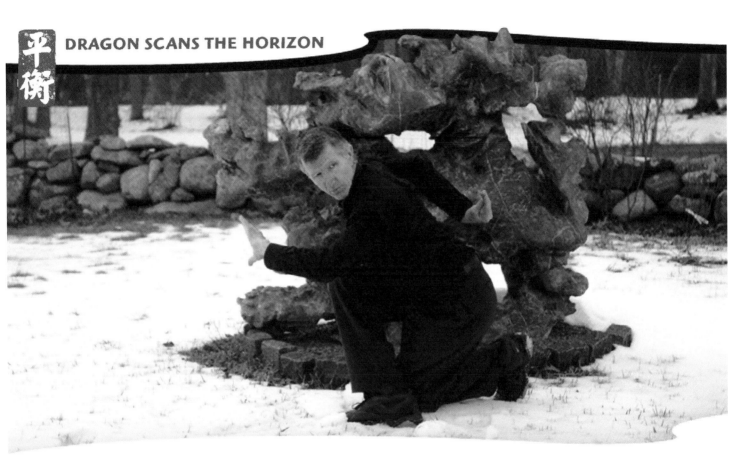

In Tai Chi, the "Dragon" refers to the twisting and turning motions made with the body, usually in support of the turning of the head and neck, as when we change the direction of our gaze. Learning to turn the head correctly, supported by a rooted stance and a flexible torso, is an essential component of good balance. The following exercise is the beginning version of Tai Chi Dragon exercises, suitable for all levels. In the photo above, Ted Box of Martha's Vineyard Tai Chi beautifully demonstrates a more advanced version of Dragon Twisting.

Start with your feet a little wider than shoulder width, weight equally distributed on both feet. Feel that your stance is firm, and rooted into the ground.

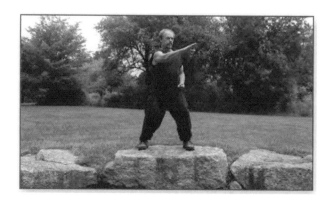

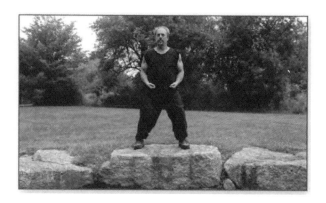

Slowly, sweep your hand across the horizon from left to right, looking where your finger points and allowing your trunk to twist gently in the direction of your gaze. Keep your feet firmly planted and make sure the legs remain firm; the head and trunk twist, but the legs do not.

Raise your right hand and point with one or two fingers at a spot on the wall (if inside) or an object or point on the visual horizon (if outside) that is the left corner of your visual field — that is, "Northwest" if you are facing north, or 10.30 if you are at the center of an imaginary clock face, facing 12. Your left hand rests at your hip, in a lightly closed fist.

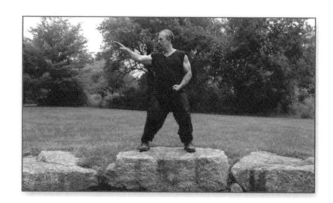

When your hand and gaze reach the right hand corner ("Northeast"), bring the hand in toward your body, closing the fingers into a light fist. Rest this hand on your hip and now extend the left hand to the right corner, pointing and gazing at the same point.

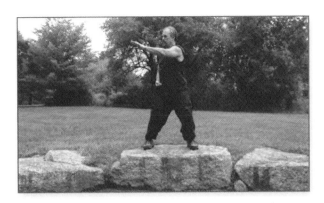

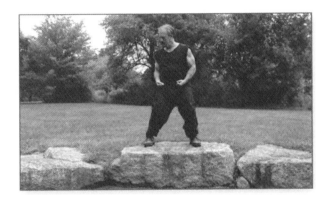

This is a complex exercise but once mastered, confers enormous benefits. Maintaining your balance as your eyes move is a critically important skill!

Pay attention to your legs, your stance, your balance, even as you are changing your gaze and your upper body position.

Slowly repeat the sweep, now going from right to left. Change hands, repeat once or twice more.

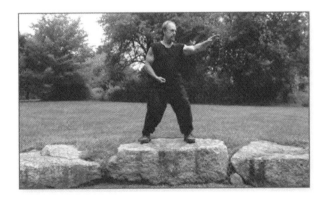

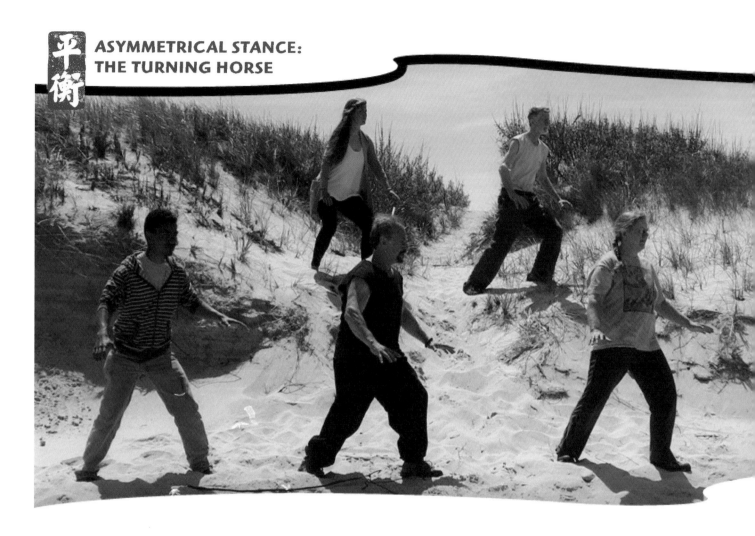

The asymmetrical stance called the "Turning Horse" is, in essence, the midpoint in the act of stepping or shifting from one foot to the other. It forms the "bridge" between standing and moving, and is an essential basic practice for developing better balance in motion.

Place one foot forward, approximately the length of a medium walking step. The angle between the feet should be approximately 45 degrees. As in all Tai Chi exercises, keep both knees slightly bent. Try to keep your weight roughly centered between front and back feet.

Your hands and arms can be either hanging loose and relaxed, or slightly opened and held away from the body (see illustration). But do not hold the arms way out to the sides and use them for balance, as a tightrope walker might do.

This is a challenging position. Maintain for as long as is comfortable, then change sides. With a rest — either in the Wu Chi position or sitting down — you can repeat on each side 3-5 times for 30 seconds to 1 minute or more. Finish in the Wu Chi posture and note the effects.

Extra Challenge: Adopt the Turning Horse stance and, once you are comfortable, try closing your eyes. You can start with just a few seconds at a time, working up to 30 seconds on each side.

When this exercise, and the others in Level One, are no longer difficult, you can progress to Level Two.

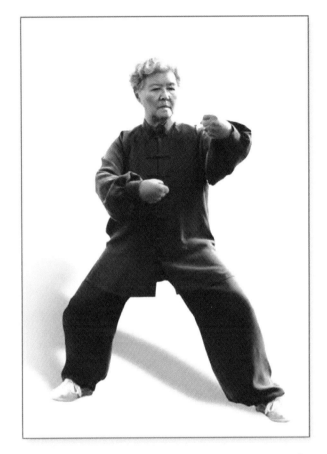

The late Madame Gao Fu, master of Chen and Yang styles of Tai Chi, displaying perfect form in the Turning Horse stance.

Tai Chi Balance Training

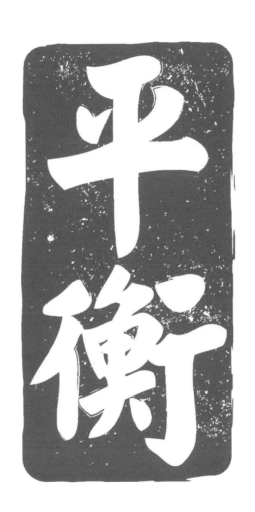

Level Two

SHIFTING WEIGHT

Shifting weight is, for many people, where their balance problems begin. Neurologically, maintaining equilibrium as you propel the body through space is infinitely more complex than maintaining equilibrium in a static position. But many people make this task even more difficult by the way in which they shift:

Balance loss frequently occurs when our head and/or upper torso are the "origin points" of the movement, such that by the time the brain registers that the weight of the upper portion has shifted, it is already at or beyond the limits of the base of support, and our balance is in jeopardy.

The Tai Chi exercises of the Five Movement Centers directly address, and resolve this problem.

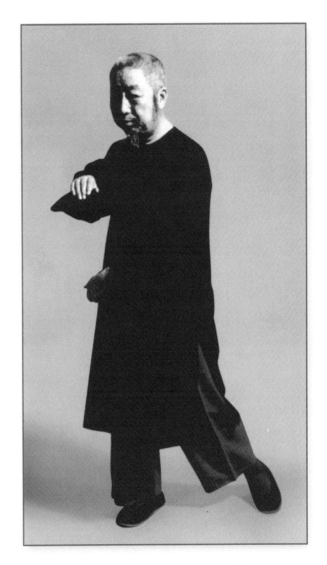

Cheng Man Ching: perfect balance (and poetry) in motion.

THE FIVE MOVEMENT CENTERS

To begin, we are going to practice moving from a variety of places in the body. Allow yourself to experience each of these fully, and note the difference in each method. Later, we will combine some of these together and see if this results in better function; but first, let's see what the possibilities are.

In each variation, try to "locate" yourself in, or focus on, the designated point or area of the body, and when you move, to move from that point or area, allowing it to "lead" the movement of the rest of the body.

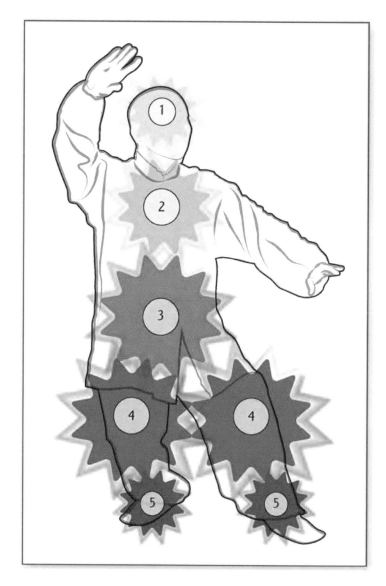

1. The Head and Face

Movement originates from the entire head, or can be localized to: the top of the head; the forehead and face; or between the eyebrows.

2. The Chest/Heart Center

Movement is now generated from the upper torso, or more specifically the center of the chest, or Emotional Center.

3. The Belly/Hips Area

In Tai Chi, an area just below the navel is referred to as the Lower Dantien, or often simply The Dantien. We can initiate movement from this specific point, or from the larger general area the includes the hips, the lower torso, groin, and buttocks.

4. The Legs

Feeling the entire mass of both legs, from hips to ankles, we move from the legs. Alternatively, we can focus separately on, and move from, the thighs; the knees; and the calves.

5. The Feet and Ankles

Now the weight is shifted by changing pressure in the ankles and feet. We can also focus more specifically on: the ankle joints; the soles of the feet; or, for a more advanced Tai Chi rooting exercise, the area just below the feet.

We will first practice moving from each of the 5 Movement Locations/Centers, while standing in a basic feet-parallel stance (Wu Chi Stance), shifting from side to side.

After we have completed the entire process in the Wu Chi stance, we will progress (at your own pace, but preferably after several sessions of the first version) to the Turning Horse asymmetrical stance, shifting the weight forward and back.

In each instance, select a Movement Center (or subcenter), and shift, at a slow to medium speed from one foot to the other, for 30 seconds to one minute.

Note the vastly differing feelings, both of physical balance and of psychological/emotional qualities, associated with each location of movement.

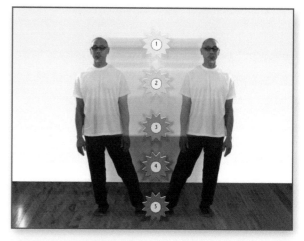

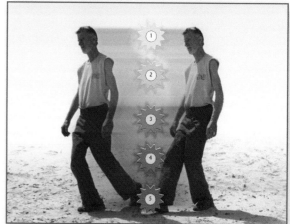

After you have completed Moving from 1 through 5, take a few seconds of stillness, then move without deliberately thinking about any specific area. See how your movement feels. How has it changed from your usual way of shifting?

COMBINING MOVEMENT CENTERS

The next step is extremely interesting: Take 2 different Movement Centers and move from both simultaneously.

Try the following combinations: 2 and 4 (Chest and Legs); 1 and 5 (Head and Feet); 3 and 5 (Hips and Feet); 2 and 3 (Chest and Hips)

Then try: 1, 3, and 5 (Head, Hips, Feet) or 2,3, and 4 (Chest, Hips, Legs). Then: 1,2,3,4 and 5 simultaneously. Then: No specific area of focus, but with all Centers activated.

There is always individual variation from person to person, but as a general Tai Chi principle, Centers 1 and 2 are considered Yang (more Up) while Centers 4 and 5 are considered Yin (more Down). Center 3 is considered to be a mixed point, where Yin and Yang meet--although it is perhaps a bit more Yin than Yang, in keeping with the Tai Chi "bias" toward the earth and nature.

Therefore, moving from Centers 1 or 2 must always be balanced by at least one from Centers 3, 4, or 5.

If you move from only one Center, it should be 3, 4, or 5.

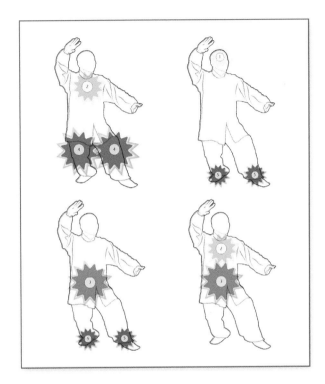

Experiment with this, test it out, observe yourself when you are moving unconsciously and see which Centers are most active, work to balance upper and lower, and pay special attention to 3 — the lower belly/hips area, which corresponds to your approximate center of gravity, and in Tai Ch is called the Lower Tan Tien. It holds the key to balance within movement.

ADVANCED SINGLE WEIGHTING

We now continue the process of strengthening the legs and deepening the root , with 3 more Single Weighted Exercises.

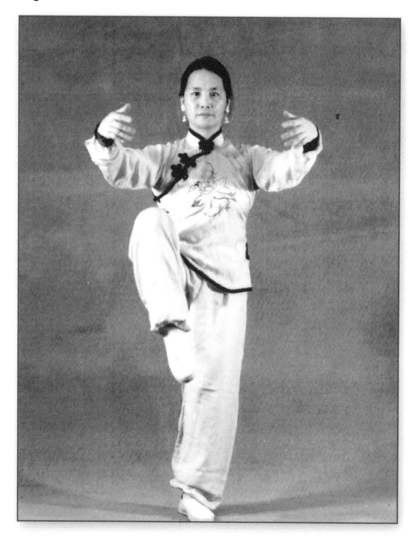

Master Bow Sim Mark, renowned and beloved teacher of authentic internal martial arts in the Boston area.

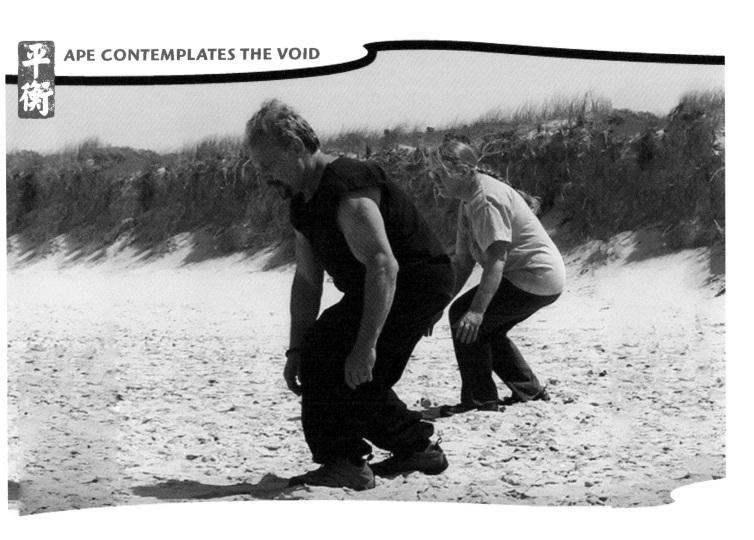

This exercise produces an almost-immediate increase in the feeling of being connected to the ground, like a tree with strong roots extending deep into the earth. You do not have to practice for many years to get this effect. Try it right now, and see.

- From a normal standing position, shift all the weight to one leg, and move the unweighted foot back 2-6 inches.

- Lift the heel of that foot off the ground, keeping contact through the ball and toes.

- Slowly sink your weight several inches by bending both at the hip joint and the knee.

NOTE: Please do not lower your body by just bending the knee, as this puts excessive strain on the knee joint and makes your much more susceptible to mis-alignments of the leg that can be both painful and damaging.

- Stop and hold the lowered position, leaving your arms loose, relaxing your back and neck as much as possible. Breathe. Your leg and hip muscles will be working, but you should not feel pain in your knee.

- Maintain this position, initially for just 30 seconds or so; then slowly stand up, without taking the weight off the foot. Pause for a few moments, feeling the muscular/energetic changes in an upright position.

- Now, bring the rear foot up and return to a parallel stance. Slowly shift your weight to the other foot, place the unweighted foot a few

inches back, sink down on the front leg (again, only a few inches or whatever is comfortable), and hold the posture again.

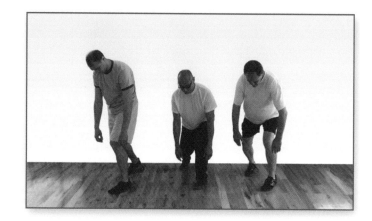

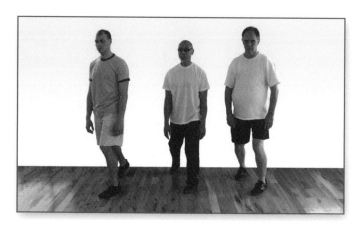

- When the second leg is "cooked," slowly rise and bring feet to parallel. And stand.

How do you feel standing now, as opposed to before the exercise? If you are like most people, you will feel quite different — legs perhaps heavy, stance more stable, as if you were connected into the earth, upper body free-er and more relaxed. Welcome to Tai Chi rooting!

As you progress, you can do 2, 3, or more "rounds" of the Ape Contemplates the Void exercise (equal time on both legs, please); and you can extend the length of time you spend in the stance each round. If you can do 3 rounds of 1 minute on each side, or a single round of 2-3 minutes (each side), comfortably, you will have made a significant beginning in developing root, strengthening your legs, and improving your stability.

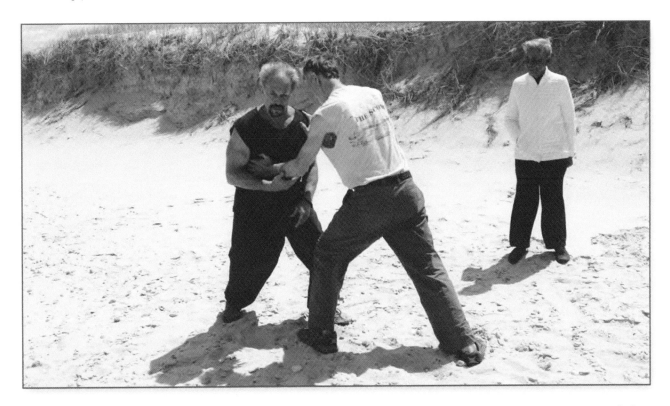

In a Two-Person Tai Chi Rooting exercise, Don "receives" Ted's push into his rear leg, maintaining stability in response to an outside force.

平衡 UNIVERSAL POST WITH EYES CLOSED

The single-weighted posture "Universal Post" from Level One can now be practiced with your eyes closed. Begin with eyes open, get stable and strong, then slowly close your eyes and allow your legs and trunk to "pick up the slack" of balancing that your vision was previously providing. If you feel at all wobbly or insecure, simply open your eyes, and relax. When you are comfortable, try again. Work up to a solid minute on each side. At this level, please open your eyes gently before you are going to change sides; later you will be able to make the change with eyes closed as well.

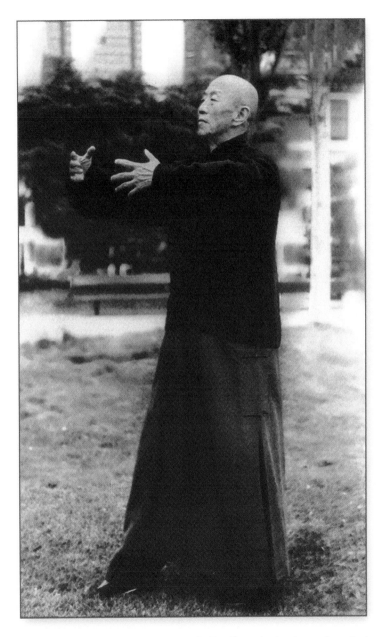

The legendary Guo Lien Ying, who taught Tai Chi and other internal arts in the San Francisco area for many years, whose personal practice included holding this posture for an hour every day.

SHIFT TO LIFTING FOOT

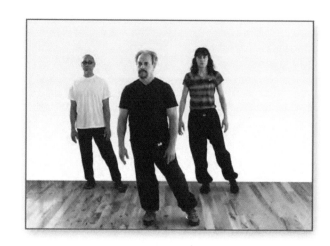

As with the Shifting Weight exercises above, we will practice this first in the Parallel (Wu Chi) stance and then in the Asymmetrical (Turning Horse) stance. Please use what you have learned about the 5 Centers to give yourself the greatest amount of stability and balance-in-motion. (If in doubt, review the "1-3-5" Combination — it works well for almost everything!)

- Starting with the parallel stance, shift your weight gradually from one leg to the other.

- As you reach almost complete single-weighting, allow the heel of the unweighted foot to come off the ground, until just ball of foot and toes are lightly touching.

- Repeat to the other side.

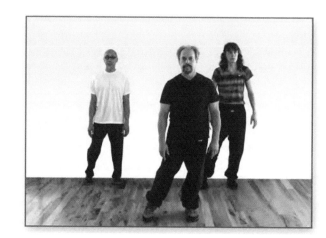

When you are comfortable with this, continue a little further and allow the unweighted heel to come off the ground, and then, let the ball and then the toes float upwards until they are an inch or so off the ground; then SOFTLY re-touch toes, then sole and heel, then resume the shift to the other side.

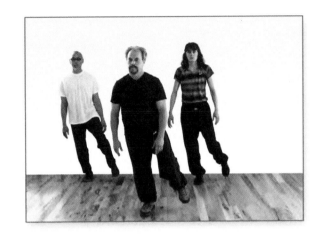

Over several sessions (take as many as you need) you will become more and more comfortable with the moments when the unweighted foot is suspended just above the ground. As you progress, you may extend the time you keep the foot up, from just a second at the beginning, to 3-5 Seconds or more. A good standard is to take one long, deep breath — inhale and exhale — with one foot off the ground, placing it down before the end of the exhale. Make sure you are always comfortable, always rooted on the supporting leg, and not struggling to hold balance. Over time, your body will get used to this and it will eventually become easy.

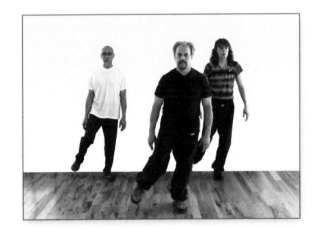

Then, progress to the same exercise in the Turning Horse Stance:

In this stance, the weight-shifting is now forward and back as opposed to side to side. Start with a shorter-than-normal stance, with only 6-12 inches' distance between your feet. (Over time, you can lengthen the stance somewhat.) When moving towards 100% single weight on the forward leg, you will lift the heel first and then the ball and toes, pretty much in the same pattern as in the Parallel stance.

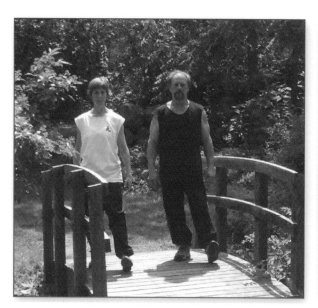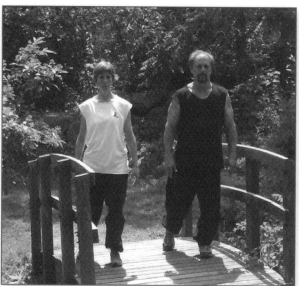

When shifting to the rear leg, the toes will come off the ground first, and the heel will be the last point of contact before the (front) foot leaves the ground.

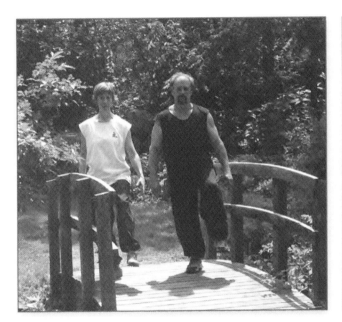 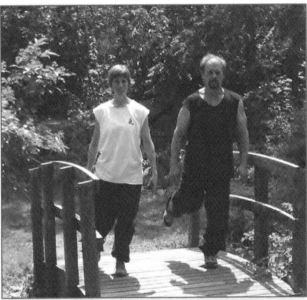

Spend enough time with this exercise so that it becomes easy and even enjoyable. Practicing "Shift and Lift" for a minute or two — involving 10-20 lifts of the foot — should become a minimum daily regime at this stage of your training. The benefits to your balance will be great!

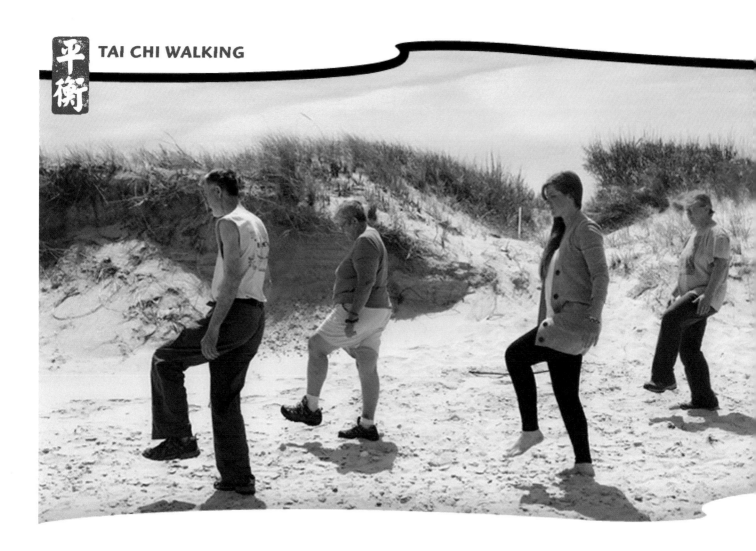

We now come to the most famous, and most important Tai Chi Balance practice, variously called Cat Stepping, Silent Walking, or Soft Stepping, but most commonly simply called Tai Chi Walking.

The basic idea is, to walk at a slow pace (one half normal walking speed, or slower); touching the ground lightly with each step before committing any weight.

There are other components of the exercise but let's begin:

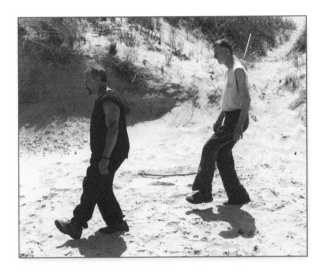 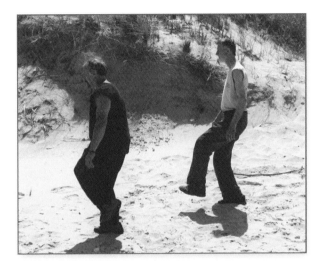

1. From a standing position, shift all the weight to one foot, and lift the other foot off the ground. Bring the unweighted foot in towards your weighted leg, and then, in an arcing pattern, take a small step forward, touching the ground lightly with your heel. Do not commit any of your body weight over the foot yet.

2. Withdraw the foot back towards the supporting leg, as a cat might do when it feels the ground is wet under a front paw. Then place the heel again, still with no weight on it.

3. Very gradually, shift weight from back foot to front foot, keeping the tai chi principles we have learned in previous shifting exercises.

4. Gradually lift the rear foot and, slowly, bring it in towards the supporting leg, then forward in a new "cat step." Touch the heel lightly. You may withdraw the foot once or twice, or proceed to slowly and gently shift the weight to this foot.

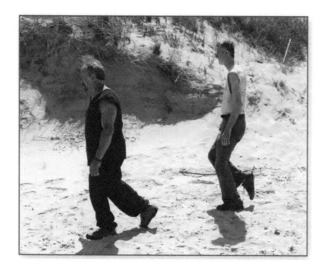 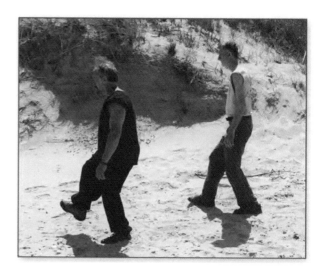

Continue walking in this manner for 10 steps or more, remembering to BREATHE, and to keep your upper body as relaxed as possible. Try not to use your arms to help you balance. They can hang loosely or be held lightly out to the sides.

Do not expect to take steps as long as your normal walking stride at first. It is far more important to remain in good balance, with root and central equilibrium, and without any feeling of "falling" onto the stepping foot. This is the major, critical difference between Tai Chi walking and normal walking.

After practicing Tai Chi Walking for a minute or more, stop and stand in the Wu Chi posture for at least a few breaths. Now return to your normal walking for a minute or so. What has changed?

When you can perform Tai Chi Walking comfortably for a minute or longer, you are ready to proceed to Level 3. But Tai Chi Walking (in this and more advanced versions) should remain a staple of your daily balance training. Tai Chi masters continue to practice this exercise for their entire lives, and as we have seen, often maintain youthful mobility, balance, and high level lower-body function into their 80's and beyond!

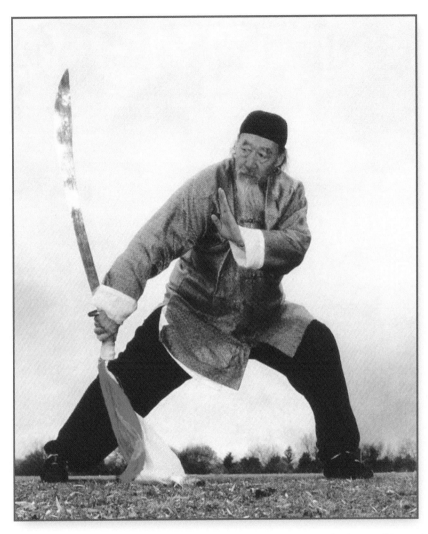

Duan Zhiliang of Beijing, an extraordinary master of qigong, martial arts, healing, and humanity.

Tai Chi Balance Training

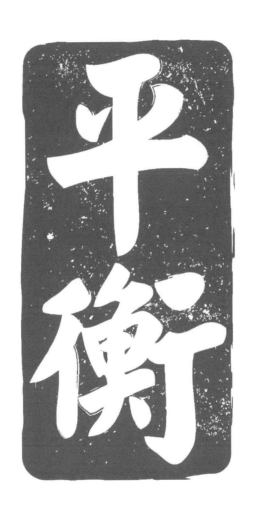

Level Three

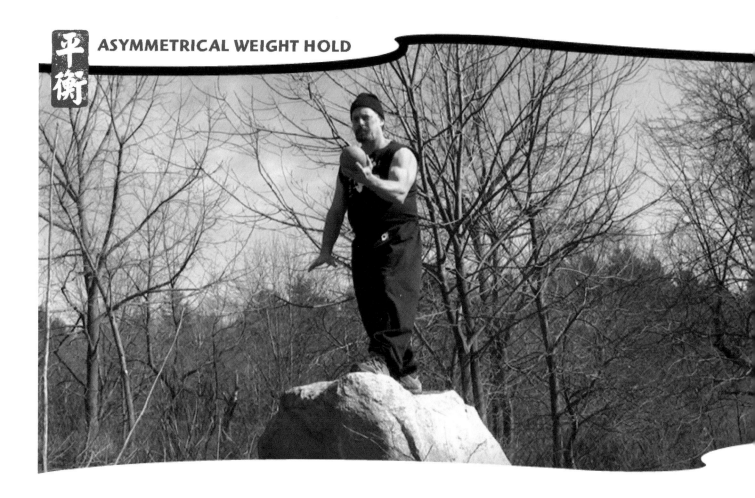

This exercise works very rapidly to give you the sense of having a strong centerline, like a tent pole with guy-wires supporting it on either side. This is the Tai Chi quality called Zhong Ding, or Central Equilibrium. In daily life we move, carry, hold, catch, and transfer objects of varying sizes and weights, and these pose a unique type of challenge to our equilibrium, as the body has to adapt to an additional weight outside itself. You will need a moderately heavy object, such as a dumbbell weight or suitcase weighing between 10 and 50 pounds.

- Stand in a parallel stance, bend from hips and knees, and lift a loaded suitcase or kettlebell or dumbbell with one hand, SLOWLY moving it from the floor (or whatever surface it rests on) to an upright standing position, with the weight as close to your body as possible. Try to stand straight, and do not lean the body either away from or on the same side as the weight.

- Pause, standing upright, and breathe for several long breaths, trying to get your body to adjust to the weight and become as comfortable as possible. Feel your feet, your legs, your trunk, the top of your head. Become stable in an upright, balanced posture, with the added weight.

- Repeat the same process with your other hand, bringing the weight to the opposite side of your body. Remember to take several breaths to accommodate the weight and stabilize your body while holding it close to you.

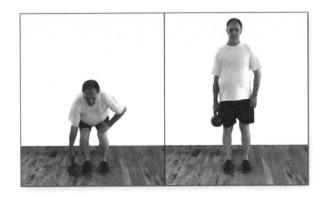

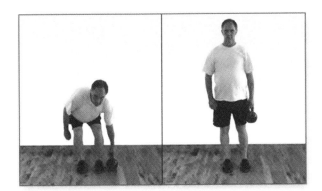

- SLOWLY fold and lower the weight to the ground.

- Stand and return to the parallel stance.

- Slowly put down the weight and stand up. Note how you feel now.

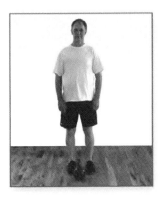

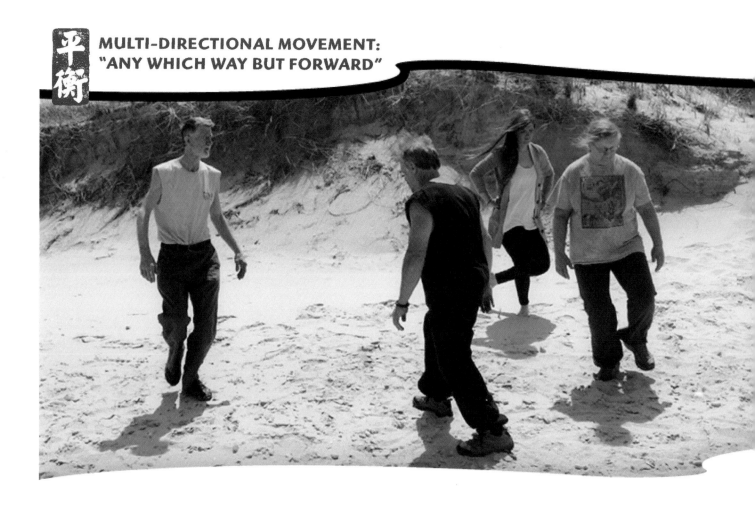

MULTI-DIRECTIONAL MOVEMENT: "ANY WHICH WAY BUT FORWARD"

This is a remarkably effective exercise for improving your balance while negotiating changes of direction, terrain, and adapting to situations that may occur while you are in motion. You will need (at first) a large, open, flat area, at least 10-15 foot square. Later you can progress to uneven surfaces or rooms with obstacles, etc, but please begin in an open, easily negotiable space.

Start walking forward at a normal pace but, within 2-3 steps, CHANGE direction by moving backwards, sideways, or at any angle except straight ahead. Continue to walk but with an almost constant series of changes — backwards for a couple of steps, then sideways, then reverse direction sideways, then move in a half-circle, then forwards, circle the other way, etc. DO NOT continue in any single pattern or direction for more than a few steps! You may stop momentarily as you change directions, but only for a moment. The important thing is to keep your feet moving in complex patterns, while maintaining balance, equilibrium, and a relaxed upright posture. Start with only 15-30 seconds, balanced by resting — in the Wu Chi stance, or, if you prefer, by walking normally in a forward direction.

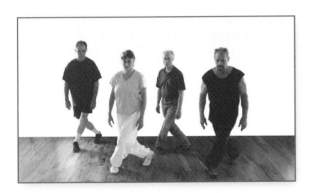
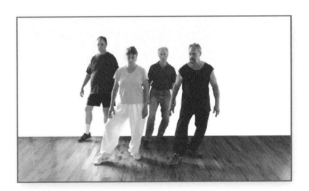
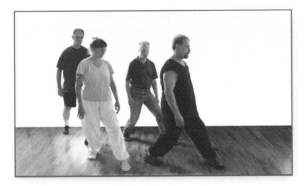
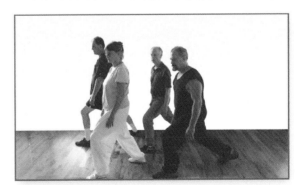

Repeat several times, as comfortable. Work up to being able to move continuously in random patterns with plenty of direction changes for 2 minutes or longer. When you can do this comfortably, you are much more likely to maintain your balance even when situations occur that demand a rapid stop or change. Good work!

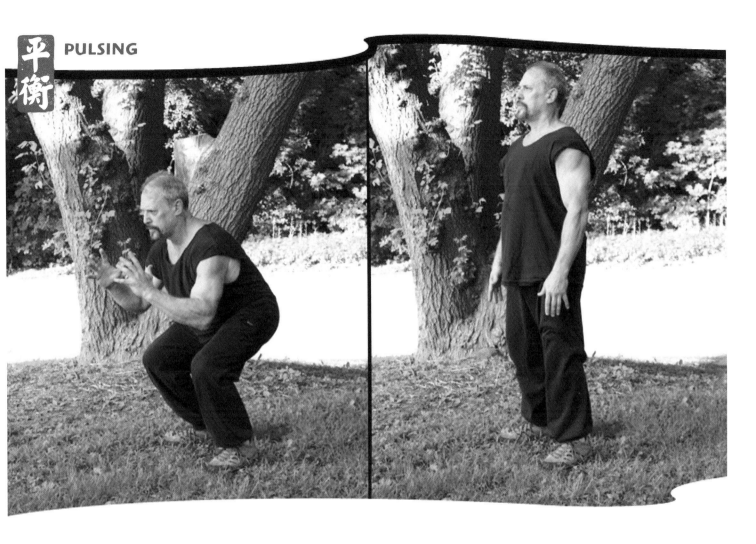

In Tai Chi, "pulsing" refers to the movement between two poles, two opposite positions or qualities — a Yin and a Yang. These could be Up and Down, Round and Straight, Heavy and Light, Coiled and Uncoiled, Drawing In and Extending Out, etc.

In this exercise, we learn to maintain Zhong Ding (central equilibrium), even when the body is moving up and down, and changing from a straight vertical position to one that is folded at key joints (hips, knees, ankles), and back again.

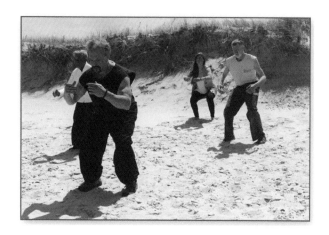
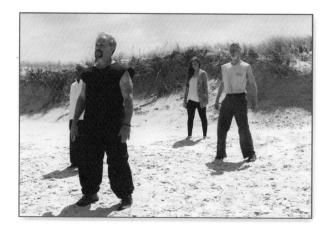

- Start in the Wu Chi parallel stance. Slowly, lower your center of gravity by bending at the hips and knees, as if you were going to sit onto a high chair. Remain aware of the soles of your feet, monitoring them closely to make sure your weight does not shift significantly backwards or forwards as you fold.

- After descending anywhere from 1–3 or more inches, slowly stand up, again making sure your weight remains on the same part of the feet.

- As you repeat the exercise for 3 to 10 repetitions or more, try to simultaneously maintain awareness of both the top of your head and the soles of the feet — or, per our previous numbering, Centers 1 and 5.

- After becoming comfortable in the parallel stance, repeat the exercise in the Turning Horse stance. Allow your body to naturally fold — like a crouching tiger — and then straighten. Repeat on both sides.

- For a greater challenge, try the up-down pulsing in the single-weighted Ape Contemplates the Void stance. This is both a great leg strengthener and rooting exercise, as well as a balance test. Just be sure your leg alignment is correct so there is no torsion or stress on the knee joint.

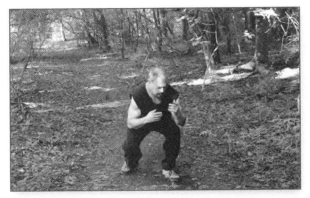

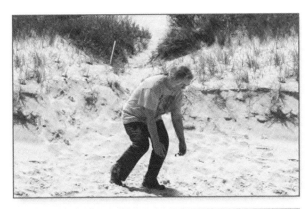

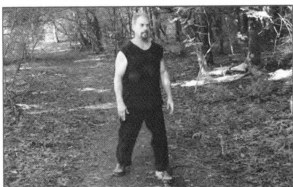

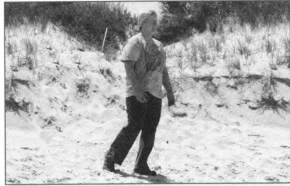

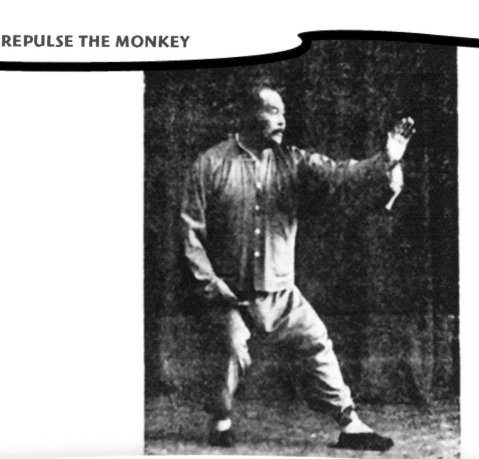

In the photo above, the legendary Yang Cheng Fu exemplifies root, central equilibrium, and energy-projection in the Yang Family version of "Step Back And Repulse The Monkey". This is a classic "form" found in all styles of Tai Chi, which teaches us to step backward without losing root or power. It trains us to withdraw from something — whether a wildly attacking "monkey-style" Kung Fu man, or a suddenly-appearing bicycle when we're out walking — without losing our balance or falling backwards.

- Start in Wu Chi.

- Shift all the weight to one foot. Sink down slightly (folding at hip and knee, as per the Pulsing exercises above) and step back with the unweighted foot, touching the ground lightly with the toes.

- Staying at the same level, gradually shift the weight to the rear foot.

- Stand up about three quarters of the way, extending your front hand (the one opposite to the leg you are standing on) in a "Stop!" gesture.

- Relax the front arm, bring it in towards your body, as you bring the unweighted front foot in towards your standing leg, and sink down (folding hip and knee) again.

- Step back lightly, shift, stand up and repeat the "Stop!" gesture with the other hand.

- Repeat on each side 5 or more times.

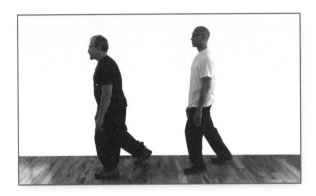

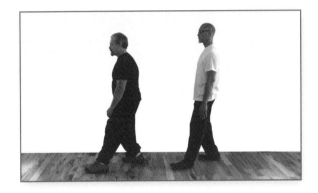

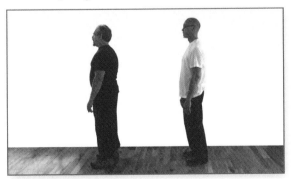

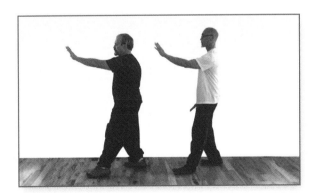

CHAIR MOVE AND SIT

Ideally, select a medium-weight chair that is easy to grasp with both hands.

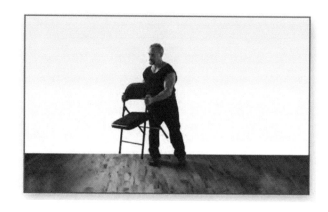

- Stand with a chair positioned about 45 degrees to the side of you.

- Maintaining root, body awareness, central equilibrium, and relaxation, lift the chair from a position on one side of your body and smoothly transfer it to the other side and set it down.

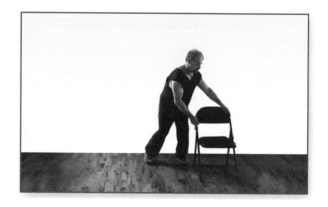

- Stand up, pause, repeat in the other direction. Pay attention to maintaining your balance and adapting to the changing position of the chair.

- Repeat several times, then place the chair down, stand for a few moments, then sit, back straight, feet apart.

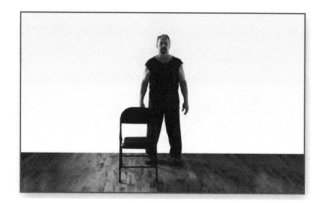

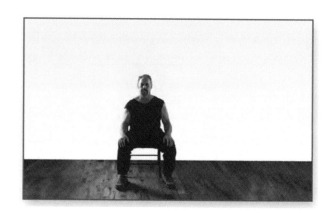

Now, you may sit in the chair and rest — or even better, practice a few minutes of:

TAOIST SITTING MEDITATION

• Feet flat on the floor, sitting close to the edge of the chair, back straight (not leaning against the back of the chair), hands resting on your thighs or in your lap.

• Half-close your eyes, breathe deeply, relax as much as possible while maintaining awareness of your body, your breath, your aliveness, the space around you (don't "zone out" or go to sleep). Empty your mind of thoughts, but remain awake and aware. If you like, you may smile inwardly. Experience stillness.

After a minute or so, you should feel calm and refreshed, physically balanced, and mentally clear.

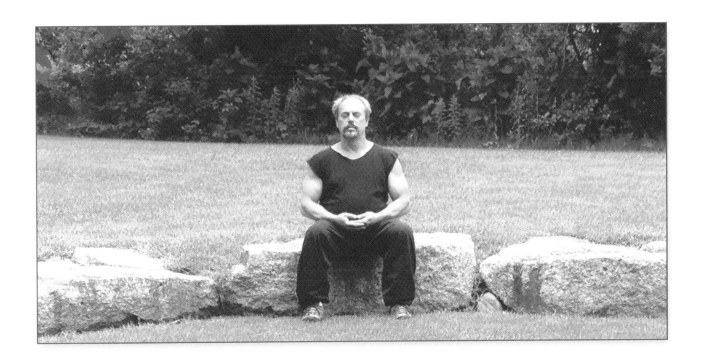

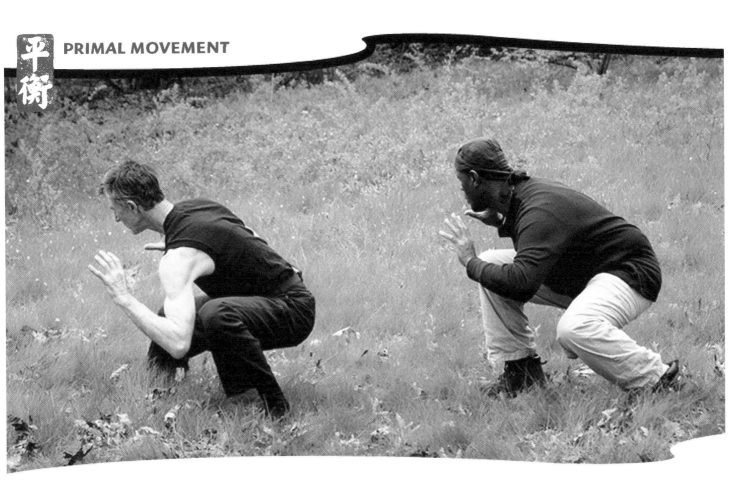

Tai Chi, and other Chinese energy-arts, frequently invoke "animal" attributes that practitioners are instructed to study and embody at certain times: the power and grace of the Tiger, the lightness and balance of the Crane, the agility and creativity of the Monkey; and many others. The final exercise of this level combines many of the things we have worked on in a single, powerful practice, adding the energies and qualities of the animal realm, and the all-important opportunity for self-expression.

We are going to move, slowly and not-so-slowly, maintaining our connection to the ground, our feeling of balance-in-motion.

We step softly, never falling onto the stepping foot.

We crouch like a tiger, rise up on one leg like a crane, move with the rooted power of the bear, the agility of the monkey, the twisting power of the dragon.

Our hands feel the air, moving in arcs and circles around the body.

We balance the Yang of Movement with the Yin of Stillness, the Yang of Intention with the Yin of Awareness.

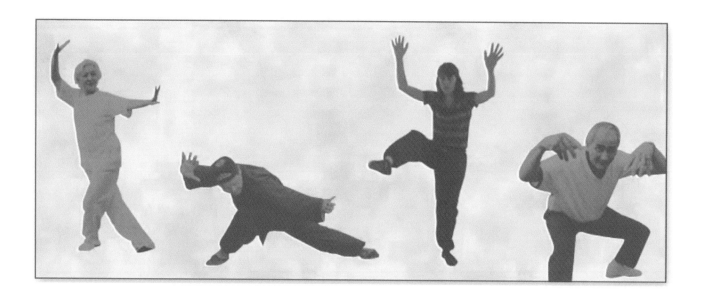

We activate all 5 Movement Centers, energizing feet and legs, head, arms, chest, waist and hips in a dynamic integrated whole.

For several minutes, we "return to nature" to dance the ancient dance, the animal dance, the primal expression of life force in posture, gesture, and action.

And then, gradually, we come to stillness in an dynamic posture, a calmness that contains all the energies and animals and powers within it. A state of profound aliveness.

We have "Entered the Gate" of Tai Chi.

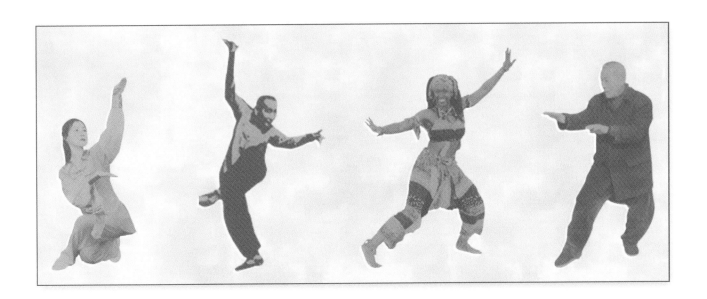

CLOSING: WU CHI

When you have finished your Tai Chi for Balance practice — whether it is just a few minutes or an hour or more — it is important to spend a few moments in the Wu Chi Standing position. Wu Chi is the empty vessel, into which we place all the energy-processes and activations we have practiced, so they will "stick" in our nervous systems and become part of us. (One of my students calls this "saving to disk".)

Once again we stand with feet roughly parallel, knees slightly bent to maintain the feeling of root, arms down or held gently in front of your torso, or hands over the dan tien, the lower abdomen.

Relax, with eyes closed or half-closed, and breathe. Let your mind be empty of thoughts, but filled with awareness. Listen to the air around you. Just stand, breathe, be aware.

Spend a minute or so in this state, enjoying the stillness that contains all movement.

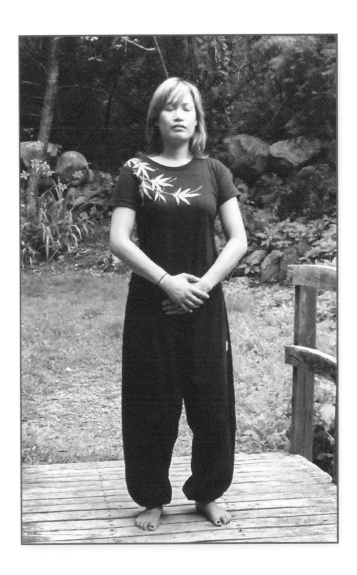

"To return to the root is to find peace."
- Lao Tzu

CONTINUING

By now, if you have progressed through the 3 Levels of Tai Chi Balance Training, and can do Level 3 comfortably, you are undoubtedly enjoying the fruits of your practice: better balance, more "root," a sense of calm power and relaxed confidence, and equilibrium in a wide variety of positions and movements. There are many different ways to continue your progress from here:

Continue to practice the exercises in this book, making them more challenging by extending times, increasing repetitions, or adding additional challenges — eyes closed, holding objects or weights, navigating uneven terrain or spaces with obstacles.

Begin (if you have not already) to study Tai Chi or related arts such as Yiquan, Bagua, and Xingyi, that share similar methods for developing root, mobility, lower body power, and equilibrium.

Challenge yourself with a new movement discipline, or revisit one that you may have practiced earlier: all forms of dance, yoga, gymnastics, athletic conditioning, ball sports, etc involve complex balance challenges and, if taken up gradually and carefully, can provide tremendous benefits to your overall well-being as well as demanding new levels of balance and coordination.

Share what you learned so far with other persons who are in need of balance improvement. By teaching the exercises, you will deepen your own understanding of the processes involved and help others at the same time. What could be better than that?

And remember, in the words of the wise T.T. Liang: "After you learn something, you must gradually change it to your own way. Blind followers are dead. Rebels can get something."

Please do not hesitate to contact us with questions, observations, suggestions, and reports on your experiences. This is, like all things, a work in progress.

Wishing you luck, laughter and great discoveries on your Tai Chi for Balance Journey!

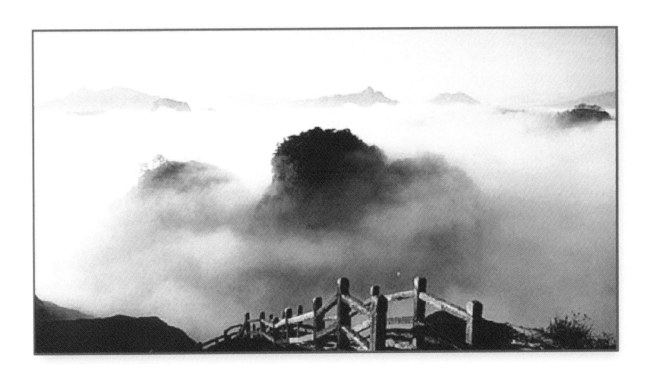

ENHANCE YOUR PRACTICE

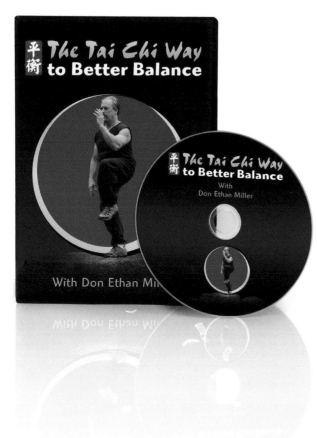

Now it's easy to work on all the exercises from the Tai Chi Way to Better Balance.

On the Tai Chi Way to Better Balance DVD, you will find practice sessions for each level of Balance Training.

Follow along with Don as you deepen your Root, challenge your Balance and find your Flow.

Visit DanKleiman.com/Balance-DVD to purchase your copy.

SPECIAL THANKS

We'd like to extend a special thanks to our teachers and fellow practitioners. If you're looking for great Tai Chi resources, check out them out.

Brookline Tai Chi: BrooklineTaiChi.org

Bruce Frantzis: EnergyArts.com

Yang Fukui: XinYiMartialArts.com

Arthur Goodridge: ArthurGoodridge.com

Hong Yijiao: ChineseWuShuTaiChi.com

Bow Sim Mark: TaiChi-Arts.com

Tung Hu Ling: DongTaiChi.com

Cheng Man Ching: ChengManChing.com

You can find Don and Dan online too:

For more of Don's DVDs on Tai Chi and other martial arts, visit MastodonProductions.com.

Dan writes, podcasts, and posts videos about Tai Chi, qigong, and movement at DanKleiman.com.

CPSIA information can be obtained at www.ICGtesting.com
Printed in the USA
LVIW01n0229040815
448750LV00006B/32